THIS BOOK BELONGS TO

This book is dedicated to those I am most grateful for,

my four daughters, Olivia, Eve, Tessa and Scarlett.

Being your mother is the greatest gift of all.

Printed in the United States of America
Second Edition, 2019
Four Little Birds Publishing

vickeryandco.com

ISBN 978-1-7336185-2-6

Cover design *by* Isabel Bogarin
Layout & typesetting *by* Jessie Leiber
Copyediting *by* Lee Lee McKnight

All quotes are used with permission of the original author

Introduction

"Remember always to marvel
at the unrelenting blessings
of your little life."

- CASEE MARIE

Journey to Gratitude

Several years ago I found myself in a very unhappy place. I was a decade into a failing marriage and I had completely lost myself. Allowing myself to stay in that unhappy space was an unintentional declaration that I deserved to be miserable, punished, and sad.

One morning at the breakfast table, I looked at each of my daughters' little faces. I wondered what their lives would be like. I thought about what I wanted for them and I imagined what I would say to them, if they were in the situation I was in: denying my true self, hiding from the world, and stuck in an unhappy, unfulfilling life.

At that very moment I knew I *wanted* to create a change. If I wanted *more* for my daughters, I had to *be* more — for myself and for them. It was time to show them that we can face challenges head-on. I knew it was important to model courageous and brave choices. And I was ready.

This decision started me on a truly transformational journey. I learned about manifestation and mindset, and, most importantly, I uncovered and embraced the power of acknowledging and expressing gratitude.

What is Gratitude?

Gratitude is a true celebration of the present: a reminder to participate fully in our lives in every possible way. It's about being aware of that which surrounds you and recognizing the gifts, large and small, even in times of difficulty. This small shift in perception can take you from a scarcity mindset to one of abundance, allowing your heart, mind, and soul, to open to even greater gifts.

Providing an avenue for acknowledging the goodness in our lives, gratitude keeps us active in the present moment. It is the process of noticing goodness and expressing our appreciation. From this, we gain a deeper understanding that the source of happiness comes from within.

Gratitude also helps us connect to something bigger than ourselves. By acknowledging gratitude we must admit there is goodness in the world. We confront the reality that we are surrounded by gifts, both tangible and intangible.

Finally, gratitude connects us to people and things in our lives that we might otherwise take for granted. Being grateful reminds us that we are not on this journey alone. Feeling more connected leads to feeling more loved and experiencing a greater sense of self-worth.

The Science Behind Gratitude

As I began to learn more about the science behind gratitude, I dug deeper into the study of Positive Psychology[1]. I was thrilled to learn more about the real science behind the power of positive thinking, which can lead to gratitude.

Psychologist Robert Emmons[2] teaches us that expressing gratitude has physiological effects on our brains—improving mental, physical, and relational well-being while reducing stress, resentment, and envy. What an extraordinary truth! Being grateful has a long-lasting impact on our overall experience of happiness.

> *"The more gratitude practice you perform in daily life, the deeper the benefits go and the more profound and life-altering the benefits truly are."*
>
> - CARLA CLARK

As I deepened my gratitude practice, I discovered that when I paid attention to the positive things happening in my life, more of them appeared. I began to feel lighter and more connected with the people and things around me, and more connected to myself.

According to Psychology Today, neurologists have proven that fear and gratitude cannot reside in the brain at the same time[3]. In fact, they are completely mutually exclusive. Focusing on gratitude crowds out fear. Gratitude is the purest form of self-love: demanding nothing, costing nothing, and giving everything.

Gratitude and Connection

In re-building my life the way I wanted it to be, and in becoming the person I wanted my girls to look up to, I learned many lessons, most notably the power of asking for help and the importance of building a support system. To be successful rebuilding my life, I couldn't do it alone.

I've always been the primary care provider for my kids, from breakfast and packed lunches to drop off and pickup. When my coaching and speaking work led to traveling more often, I needed to hand off these duties.

Babysitters were expensive and not always available, so I had to ask my ex-spouse to step-up and be active in areas that had previously been my domain. I also coordinated with friends to arrange playdates for my kids after school until their father could pick them up.

These may seem like small, silly requests, but, as a woman, I'd been conditioned to see weakness in asking for help. With life's circumstances at play, I no longer had the option to believe in that myth. I had to come up with a solution so that I could travel and earn money without sacrificing my kids' care.

By simply *asking* for this support and then receiving it, I instantly felt more loved and supported—an extraordinary feeling that brought me to a new level of gratitude. A rush of emotion overcame me: I was loved and valued and worthy.

In theory, we should not need outside elements to prove we are loved, valued, and worthy, but human beings need validation. By realizing this fact, acknowledging it, and expressing gratitude to myself and those that supported me, my community relationships grew evermore deep and powerful.

Why Practice Gratitude?

Life, as complex as it is, will always include pain and challenges. However, when you ground your thoughts and actions in gratitude, you can find beauty and joy in every aspect of life.

By actively working to focus your thoughts and center them around what you have to be grateful for, you will move away from what is lacking in your life and wrap yourself in the abundance that already exists.

Many of you may be familiar with The Law Of Attraction, a thought practice that was taught by Buddha hundreds of years ago. At its core, the idea is that *what you have become is what you have thought.* In other words, thoughts become things and our perception creates our reality.[4]

In simple terms, the Law of Attraction is the ability to attract into our lives that which we focus on. The mind has the power to translate our thoughts and materialize them into reality. What you think will, eventually, become your reality.

If you focus on negative thoughts and emotions, those will appear in abundance. If you focus on gratitude you will have much more to be grateful for. This thought process opens up space to achieve your goals with massive action.

Recording experiences for which we are grateful has wide-reaching positive effects including greater alertness, more energy, and increased enthusiasm, as well as a rise in determination and attentiveness. Evidence also shows a renewed commitment to self-care and being physically fit!

Expressing Gratitude

Personally, I find much joy in expressing and sharing my gratitude with and towards others. My family and I have a ritual each night during dinner. We go around the table and share one thing we enjoyed about our day and what we are most grateful for.

Some days these things come to us easily and some days we struggle. What I especially love about this exercise is that my children are able to see that even on the most difficult of days, there is something to celebrate and something for which we can be grateful.

I also make every effort to share, on the spot, my gratitude for another person. I know firsthand the warmth and connection verbal appreciation or affirmation can bring, not to mention the validation of feeling noticed that all human beings crave.

With that in mind, I'm happy to tell you how unbelievably grateful I am to you for purchasing this journal. I encourage you to express your gratitude in a bold and brave way. In so doing, you will retrain your brain to see the wonder and possibility that is constantly ahead of you.

Heather

CITATIONS

[1] *Positive Psychology is the scientific study of the strengths that enable individuals and communities to thrive. The field is founded on the belief that people want to lead meaningful and fulfilling lives, to cultivate what is best within themselves, and to enhance their experiences of love, work, and play.*

[2] *Robert Emmons, Ph. D., is a Professor of Psychology at the University of California at Davis. His research is in the field of personality psychology, emotion psychology, and psychology of religion.*

[3] *Korb, Alex, Ph.D. (2012, Nov) The Grateful Brain. retrieved from https://www.psychologytoday.com/us/blog/prefrontal-nudity/201211/the-grateful-brain.*

[4] *For more about The Law of Attraction, I recommend starting at TheLawofAttraction.com.*

WAYS TO USE THIS
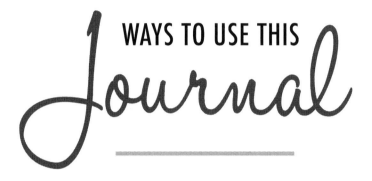
Journal

"Gratitude is the fairest blossom which springs from the soul."

- HENRY WARD BEECHER

This journal contains room for 180 separate entries. I invite and encourage you to write in it however often you want. Some people practice gratitude as a daily ritual, some journal a few times a week, and others notice gratefulness weekly. There is no right or wrong way to record your gratitude. Trust your gut.

You will also find 180 unique prompts included in this journal. Each prompt is designed to help you think creatively about your life and all that you have to be grateful for. Enjoy exploring areas you may never have even considered being grateful for in the past!

I promise you this: if you practice gratitude consistently for at least six weeks, you will discover a level of peace, understanding, and happiness that you've never encountered before. Increases in these feelings will lead to a more balanced, successful life on every level.

When sitting down to record your gratitude, you may want to reflect on these things:

- A person that has impacted you that day

- A thought that connects with you

- An action you took or someone else took

- An act of joy you have experienced or provided

Journaling is not the only way to connect with gratitude. I personally bring gratitude into my life in a multitude of ways. Here are a few suggestions. Consider adding some of these to your gratitude practices and do what feels right!

- Breathe deeply before and after your gratitude journaling. This ensures you are present, grounded, and mindful.

- Mentally acknowledge things you are grateful for in the moment, when the thought first occurs to you.

- Redirect anger or frustration by finding something to be grateful for in a frustrating moment. For example, being stuck in terrible traffic is frustrating. When I find myself in that situation, I will express gratitude for being safe in my car and not involved in a car accident.

- Express thanks, often, and to everyone you encounter!

- Write a letter of thanks to someone who has made a difference in your life.

- Have a shared family (or friend) gratitude practice.

- Go deep with your gratitude. Rather than rattling off a quick list of things, elaborate about what you are grateful for.

- Make it personal — focus on the people that impact your life. It will help you connect with those people on many levels.

- Find gratitude for little things that will help you reach big goals. Envision yourself having accomplished those goals.

START
Today

"Expressing gratitude helps me remember the magic of life."

- LATOYA BURON

TODAY I AM GRATEFUL FOR...

- My oldest child still wanting me to tuck her into bed at night and sing to her
- Listening to others laugh
- The way the sun streams through the window in the morning
- A hot cup of coffee

PERSONAL HIGH FIVES (WINS)

- Hearing from a past client that the work we did together has made a big impact on their life
- Getting the kids to school on time without morning drama
- Writing for an hour because it makes me feel grounded

HOW DID YOU EXPRESS GRATITUDE TODAY?

I thanked a co-worker for all of their hard work on a new project. They were an important part of our team success and I wanted to know how much their effort mattered to me.

WHAT CHAOS ARE YOU GRATEFUL FOR TODAY?

The hustle and bustle of making breakfast and lunches for four kids in the morning. I am grateful we have plenty of food to eat and that I have these amazing kids to keep me on my toes.

TODAY I AM GRATEFUL FOR...

PERSONAL HIGH FIVES (WINS)

HOW DID YOU EXPRESS GRATITUDE TODAY?

WHAT ELECTRONIC ARE YOU MOST GRATEFUL FOR?

TODAY I AM GRATEFUL FOR...

PERSONAL HIGH FIVES (WINS)

HOW DID YOU EXPRESS GRATITUDE TODAY?

WHAT ARE YOU MOST GRATEFUL FOR IN THE SPRING?

TODAY I AM GRATEFUL FOR...

PERSONAL HIGH FIVES (WINS)

HOW DID YOU EXPRESS GRATITUDE TODAY?

WHAT MEMORY BROUGHT YOU PLEASURE TODAY?

TODAY I AM GRATEFUL FOR...

PERSONAL HIGH FIVES (WINS)

HOW DID YOU EXPRESS GRATITUDE TODAY?

WHAT IS YOUR FAVORITE ICE CREAM FLAVOR?

TODAY I AM GRATEFUL FOR...

PERSONAL HIGH FIVES (WINS)

HOW DID YOU EXPRESS GRATITUDE TODAY?

WHAT SOUNDS ARE YOU GRATEFUL FOR TODAY?

"Reflect upon your present blessings... not on your past misfortunes."

CHARLES DICKENS

TODAY I AM GRATEFUL FOR...

PERSONAL HIGH FIVES (WINS)

HOW DID YOU EXPRESS GRATITUDE TODAY?

WHICH BODY PART ARE YOU MOST GRATEFUL FOR TODAY?

TODAY I AM GRATEFUL FOR...

PERSONAL HIGH FIVES (WINS)

HOW DID YOU EXPRESS GRATITUDE TODAY?

WHAT MEMORY ARE YOU MOST GRATEFUL FOR?

TODAY I AM GRATEFUL FOR...

PERSONAL HIGH FIVES (WINS)

HOW DID YOU EXPRESS GRATITUDE TODAY?

WHAT FOOD ARE YOU MOST GRATEFUL FOR?

TODAY I AM GRATEFUL FOR...

PERSONAL HIGH FIVES (WINS)

HOW DID YOU EXPRESS GRATITUDE TODAY?

WHAT IS THE MOST BEAUTIFUL THING YOU SAW OR EXPERIENCED TODAY?

TODAY I AM GRATEFUL FOR...

PERSONAL HIGH FIVES (WINS)

HOW DID YOU EXPRESS GRATITUDE TODAY?

WHAT UNUSUAL THING ARE YOU MOST GRATEFUL FOR?

TODAY I AM GRATEFUL FOR...

PERSONAL HIGH FIVES (WINS)

HOW DID YOU EXPRESS GRATITUDE TODAY?

WHAT MODERN INVENTION ARE YOU MOST GRATEFUL FOR?

"Be aware of your feelings and how you 'relish' and 'savor' this gift in your imagination. Take the time to be especially aware of the depth of your gratitude."

ROBERT EMMONS

TODAY I AM GRATEFUL FOR...

PERSONAL HIGH FIVES (WINS)

HOW DID YOU EXPRESS GRATITUDE TODAY?

WHAT ELEMENT OF NATURE ARE YOU MOST GRATEFUL FOR?

TODAY I AM GRATEFUL FOR...

PERSONAL HIGH FIVES (WINS)

HOW DID YOU EXPRESS GRATITUDE TODAY?

WHAT THROW BACK SMELL FROM YOUR CHILDHOOD ARE YOU GRATEFUL FOR?

TODAY I AM GRATEFUL FOR...

PERSONAL HIGH FIVES (WINS)

HOW DID YOU EXPRESS GRATITUDE TODAY?

WHAT NATURAL BODILY FUNCTION ARE YOU GRATEFUL FOR?

TODAY I AM GRATEFUL FOR...

PERSONAL HIGH FIVES (WINS)

HOW DID YOU EXPRESS GRATITUDE TODAY?

WHAT PERSON ARE YOU MOST GRATEFUL FOR TODAY?

TODAY I AM GRATEFUL FOR...

PERSONAL HIGH FIVES (WINS)

HOW DID YOU EXPRESS GRATITUDE TODAY?

WHAT HOUSEHOLD CHORE ARE YOU GRATEFUL FOR TODAY?

"Gratitude bestows reverence, allowing us to encounter everyday epiphanies, those transcendent moments of awe that change forever how we experience life and the world."

JOHN MILTON

TODAY I AM GRATEFUL FOR...

PERSONAL HIGH FIVES (WINS)

HOW DID YOU EXPRESS GRATITUDE TODAY?

WHAT MADE YOU LAUGH OUT LOUD TODAY?

TODAY I AM GRATEFUL FOR...

PERSONAL HIGH FIVES (WINS)

HOW DID YOU EXPRESS GRATITUDE TODAY?

WHAT MADE YOU JOYFUL TODAY?

TODAY I AM GRATEFUL FOR...

PERSONAL HIGH FIVES (WINS)

HOW DID YOU EXPRESS GRATITUDE TODAY?

WHAT WERE YOU ENTHUSIASTIC ABOUT TODAY?

TODAY I AM GRATEFUL FOR...

PERSONAL HIGH FIVES (WINS)

HOW DID YOU EXPRESS GRATITUDE TODAY?

WHAT FAMILY MEMBER ARE YOU MOST GRATEFUL FOR TODAY?

TODAY I AM GRATEFUL FOR...

PERSONAL HIGH FIVES (WINS)

HOW DID YOU EXPRESS GRATITUDE TODAY?

WHAT MADE YOU HOPEFUL TODAY?

TODAY I AM GRATEFUL FOR...

PERSONAL HIGH FIVES (WINS)

HOW DID YOU EXPRESS GRATITUDE TODAY?

WHICH ROOM IN YOUR HOME ARE YOU MOST GRATEFUL FOR TODAY?

"The things we use every day aren't trivial; even if they're utilitarian in nature, we can still appreciate them."

LEE LEE MCKNIGHT

TODAY I AM GRATEFUL FOR...

PERSONAL HIGH FIVES (WINS)

HOW DID YOU EXPRESS GRATITUDE TODAY?

WHAT PLEASANTLY SURPRISED YOU TODAY?

TODAY I AM GRATEFUL FOR...

PERSONAL HIGH FIVES (WINS)

HOW DID YOU EXPRESS GRATITUDE TODAY?

HOW DID YOU HELP ANOTHER PERSON TODAY?

TODAY I AM GRATEFUL FOR...

PERSONAL HIGH FIVES (WINS)

HOW DID YOU EXPRESS GRATITUDE TODAY?

WHAT KINDNESS ARE YOU GRATEFUL FOR TODAY?

TODAY I AM GRATEFUL FOR...

PERSONAL HIGH FIVES (WINS)

HOW DID YOU EXPRESS GRATITUDE TODAY?

WHAT SWEET, SIMPLE THING ARE YOU GRATEFUL FOR TODAY?

TODAY I AM GRATEFUL FOR...

PERSONAL HIGH FIVES (WINS)

HOW DID YOU EXPRESS GRATITUDE TODAY?

WHAT BRAVE THING DID YOU DO TODAY?

"You can nearly always enjoy things if you make up your mind firmly that you will."

LUCY MAUD MONTGOMERY

TODAY I AM GRATEFUL FOR...

PERSONAL HIGH FIVES (WINS)

HOW DID YOU EXPRESS GRATITUDE TODAY?

HOW DID SOMEONE COME THROUGH FOR YOU TODAY?

TODAY I AM GRATEFUL FOR...

PERSONAL HIGH FIVES (WINS)

HOW DID YOU EXPRESS GRATITUDE TODAY?

WHICH FAMILY RECIPE ARE YOU MOST GRATEFUL FOR?

TODAY I AM GRATEFUL FOR...

PERSONAL HIGH FIVES (WINS)

HOW DID YOU EXPRESS GRATITUDE TODAY?

WHAT KINDNESS DID YOU SHOW ANOTHER PERSON TODAY?

TODAY I AM GRATEFUL FOR...

PERSONAL HIGH FIVES (WINS)

HOW DID YOU EXPRESS GRATITUDE TODAY?

WHAT IS THE FUNNIEST THING YOU EXPERIENCED TODAY?

TODAY I AM GRATEFUL FOR...

PERSONAL HIGH FIVES (WINS)

HOW DID YOU EXPRESS GRATITUDE TODAY?

WHAT POSITIVE LESSON DID YOU LEARN TODAY?

TODAY I AM GRATEFUL FOR...

PERSONAL HIGH FIVES (WINS)

HOW DID YOU EXPRESS GRATITUDE TODAY?

WHAT ARE YOU MOST EXCITED ABOUT TODAY?

"Let us be grateful to people who make us happy, they are the charming gardeners who make our souls blossom."

MARCEL PROUST

TODAY I AM GRATEFUL FOR...

PERSONAL HIGH FIVES (WINS)

HOW DID YOU EXPRESS GRATITUDE TODAY?

WHAT CHANGE IS POSSIBLE TODAY?

TODAY I AM GRATEFUL FOR...

PERSONAL HIGH FIVES (WINS)

HOW DID YOU EXPRESS GRATITUDE TODAY?

WHAT ACHIEVEMENT BROUGHT YOU JOY TODAY?

TODAY I AM GRATEFUL FOR...

PERSONAL HIGH FIVES (WINS)

HOW DID YOU EXPRESS GRATITUDE TODAY?

WHAT SONG ARE YOU MOST GRATEFUL FOR?

TODAY I AM GRATEFUL FOR...

PERSONAL HIGH FIVES (WINS)

HOW DID YOU EXPRESS GRATITUDE TODAY?

WHAT DID YOU MOST ENJOY DOING TODAY?

TODAY I AM GRATEFUL FOR...

PERSONAL HIGH FIVES (WINS)

HOW DID YOU EXPRESS GRATITUDE TODAY?

HOW DID YOU MAKE YOURSELF PROUD TODAY?

"I am constantly grateful for all I have and all I don't have."

PAMELA FREESE

TODAY I AM GRATEFUL FOR...

PERSONAL HIGH FIVES (WINS)

HOW DID YOU EXPRESS GRATITUDE TODAY?

WHAT RARE PLEASURE DID YOU ENJOY TODAY?

TODAY I AM GRATEFUL FOR...

PERSONAL HIGH FIVES (WINS)

HOW DID YOU EXPRESS GRATITUDE TODAY?

WHAT SEASON ARE YOU MOST GRATEFUL FOR?

TODAY I AM GRATEFUL FOR...

PERSONAL HIGH FIVES (WINS)

HOW DID YOU EXPRESS GRATITUDE TODAY?

WHAT MADE YOU INSANELY HAPPY TODAY?

TODAY I AM GRATEFUL FOR...

PERSONAL HIGH FIVES (WINS)

HOW DID YOU EXPRESS GRATITUDE TODAY?

WHAT DID YOU HAPPILY SAY NO TO TODAY?

TODAY I AM GRATEFUL FOR...

PERSONAL HIGH FIVES (WINS)

HOW DID YOU EXPRESS GRATITUDE TODAY?

WHAT QUIET PLEASURE ARE YOU MOST GRATEFUL FOR TODAY?

TODAY I AM GRATEFUL FOR...

PERSONAL HIGH FIVES (WINS)

HOW DID YOU EXPRESS GRATITUDE TODAY?

WHAT PERSONAL HYGIENE ROUTINE ARE YOU MOST GRATEFUL FOR TODAY?

"Being grateful
every day is
something you
have to work at."

NICOLE ZENNER

TODAY I AM GRATEFUL FOR...

PERSONAL HIGH FIVES (WINS)

HOW DID YOU EXPRESS GRATITUDE TODAY?

WHAT HOLIDAY ARE YOU MOST GRATEFUL FOR?

TODAY I AM GRATEFUL FOR...

PERSONAL HIGH FIVES (WINS)

HOW DID YOU EXPRESS GRATITUDE TODAY?

WHAT DID YOU CREATE TODAY?

TODAY I AM GRATEFUL FOR...

PERSONAL HIGH FIVES (WINS)

HOW DID YOU EXPRESS GRATITUDE TODAY?

WHAT ARE YOU MOST GRATEFUL FOR ABOUT YOUR AGE?

TODAY I AM GRATEFUL FOR...

PERSONAL HIGH FIVES (WINS)

HOW DID YOU EXPRESS GRATITUDE TODAY?

WHAT FEAR DID YOU OVERCOME TODAY?

TODAY I AM GRATEFUL FOR...

PERSONAL HIGH FIVES (WINS)

HOW DID YOU EXPRESS GRATITUDE TODAY?

WHAT IS THE MOST DELICIOUS THING YOU TASTED TODAY?

"We can complain because rose bushes have thorns, or rejoice because thorns have roses."

ALPHONSE KARR

TODAY I AM GRATEFUL FOR...

PERSONAL HIGH FIVES (WINS)

HOW DID YOU EXPRESS GRATITUDE TODAY?

WHAT GAVE YOU THE MOST PLEASURE TODAY?

TODAY I AM GRATEFUL FOR...

PERSONAL HIGH FIVES (WINS)

HOW DID YOU EXPRESS GRATITUDE TODAY?

WHAT ARE YOU OPTIMISTIC ABOUT TODAY?

TODAY I AM GRATEFUL FOR...

PERSONAL HIGH FIVES (WINS)

HOW DID YOU EXPRESS GRATITUDE TODAY?

WHAT SEEMINGLY BORING TASK DO YOU ENJOY?

TODAY I AM GRATEFUL FOR...

PERSONAL HIGH FIVES (WINS)

HOW DID YOU EXPRESS GRATITUDE TODAY?

WHAT ITEM OF CLOTHING ARE YOU MOST GRATEFUL FOR TODAY?

TODAY I AM GRATEFUL FOR...

PERSONAL HIGH FIVES (WINS)

HOW DID YOU EXPRESS GRATITUDE TODAY?

WHAT ROUTINE ACTIVITY BROUGHT YOU JOY TODAY?

TODAY I AM GRATEFUL FOR...

PERSONAL HIGH FIVES (WINS)

HOW DID YOU EXPRESS GRATITUDE TODAY?

WHAT NEW THING DID YOU LEARN TODAY?

"The smallest act of
kindness is worth
more than the
grandest intention."

KAHLIL GIBRAN

TODAY I AM GRATEFUL FOR...

PERSONAL HIGH FIVES (WINS)

HOW DID YOU EXPRESS GRATITUDE TODAY?

WHAT TEDIOUS TASK ARE YOU MOST GRATEFUL FOR?

TODAY I AM GRATEFUL FOR...

PERSONAL HIGH FIVES (WINS)

HOW DID YOU EXPRESS GRATITUDE TODAY?

WHAT DID YOU MOST ENJOY DOING ALONE TODAY?

TODAY I AM GRATEFUL FOR...

PERSONAL HIGH FIVES (WINS)

HOW DID YOU EXPRESS GRATITUDE TODAY?

HOW DID YOU TREAT YOURSELF TODAY?

TODAY I AM GRATEFUL FOR...

PERSONAL HIGH FIVES (WINS)

HOW DID YOU EXPRESS GRATITUDE TODAY?

WHAT DO YOU HOPE IS POSSIBLE?

TODAY I AM GRATEFUL FOR...

PERSONAL HIGH FIVES (WINS)

HOW DID YOU EXPRESS GRATITUDE TODAY?

WHAT MAKES YOUR HEART SKIP A BEAT?

"Gratitude is the healthiest of all human emotions. The more you express gratitude for what you have, the more likely you will have even more to express gratitude for."

—

ZIG ZIGLAR

TODAY I AM GRATEFUL FOR...

PERSONAL HIGH FIVES (WINS)

HOW DID YOU EXPRESS GRATITUDE TODAY?

WHAT MOVIE COULD YOU WATCH OVER AND OVER AGAIN?

TODAY I AM GRATEFUL FOR...

PERSONAL HIGH FIVES (WINS)

HOW DID YOU EXPRESS GRATITUDE TODAY?

WHAT IS YOUR THEME SONG?

TODAY I AM GRATEFUL FOR...

PERSONAL HIGH FIVES (WINS)

HOW DID YOU EXPRESS GRATITUDE TODAY?

WHO WAS YOUR BIGGEST FAN TODAY?

TODAY I AM GRATEFUL FOR...

PERSONAL HIGH FIVES (WINS)

HOW DID YOU EXPRESS GRATITUDE TODAY?

WHICH HOLIDAY TRADITION DO YOU MOST ENJOY?

TODAY I AM GRATEFUL FOR...

PERSONAL HIGH FIVES (WINS)

HOW DID YOU EXPRESS GRATITUDE TODAY?

WHAT DESSERT ARE YOU MOST GRATEFUL FOR?

TODAY I AM GRATEFUL FOR...

PERSONAL HIGH FIVES (WINS)

HOW DID YOU EXPRESS GRATITUDE TODAY?

WHAT MEMORY MAKES YOU LAUGH UNTIL YOUR SIDE HURTS?

"Life will always
be messy, but joy
can be found in
the journey of
ups and downs."

DEVIN DONALDSON

TODAY I AM GRATEFUL FOR...

PERSONAL HIGH FIVES (WINS)

HOW DID YOU EXPRESS GRATITUDE TODAY?

WHAT DRINK ARE YOU MOST GRATEFUL FOR?

TODAY I AM GRATEFUL FOR...

PERSONAL HIGH FIVES (WINS)

HOW DID YOU EXPRESS GRATITUDE TODAY?

WHAT SEEMINGLY "USUAL" THING ARE YOU MOST GRATEFUL FOR?

TODAY I AM GRATEFUL FOR...

PERSONAL HIGH FIVES (WINS)

HOW DID YOU EXPRESS GRATITUDE TODAY?

WHAT MEMORY MOST WARMS YOUR HEART?

TODAY I AM GRATEFUL FOR...

PERSONAL HIGH FIVES (WINS)

HOW DID YOU EXPRESS GRATITUDE TODAY?

WHAT MESS ARE YOU GRATEFUL FOR?

TODAY I AM GRATEFUL FOR...

PERSONAL HIGH FIVES (WINS)

HOW DID YOU EXPRESS GRATITUDE TODAY?

WHAT CONVERSATION ARE YOU GRATEFUL FOR TODAY?

"The potential for joy exists in most of our daily actions and adventures."

MARIE LEVEY-PABST

TODAY I AM GRATEFUL FOR...

PERSONAL HIGH FIVES (WINS)

HOW DID YOU EXPRESS GRATITUDE TODAY?

WHAT PIECE OF ADVICE ARE YOU MOST GRATEFUL FOR TODAY?

TODAY I AM GRATEFUL FOR...

PERSONAL HIGH FIVES (WINS)

HOW DID YOU EXPRESS GRATITUDE TODAY?

WHAT IS THE STRANGEST THING YOU ARE GRATEFUL FOR TODAY?

TODAY I AM GRATEFUL FOR...

PERSONAL HIGH FIVES (WINS)

HOW DID YOU EXPRESS GRATITUDE TODAY?

WHAT DAILY RITUAL ARE YOU MOST GRATEFUL FOR TODAY?

TODAY I AM GRATEFUL FOR...

PERSONAL HIGH FIVES (WINS)

HOW DID YOU EXPRESS GRATITUDE TODAY?

NAME ONE PLACE YOU ARE GRATEFUL FOR HAVING VISITED.

TODAY I AM GRATEFUL FOR...

PERSONAL HIGH FIVES (WINS)

HOW DID YOU EXPRESS GRATITUDE TODAY?

HOW DID YOU EXPRESS GRATITUDE FOR ANOTHER TODAY?

TODAY I AM GRATEFUL FOR...

PERSONAL HIGH FIVES (WINS)

HOW DID YOU EXPRESS GRATITUDE TODAY?

WHAT CONNECTION ARE YOU GRATEFUL FOR TODAY?

"Gratitude is an antidote to negative emotions, a neutralizer of envy, hostility, worry, and irritation. It is savoring; it is not taking things for granted; it is present oriented."

SONJA LYUBOMIRSKY

TODAY I AM GRATEFUL FOR...

PERSONAL HIGH FIVES (WINS)

HOW DID YOU EXPRESS GRATITUDE TODAY?

WHICH HOLIDAY FOOD ARE YOU MOST GRATEFUL FOR?

TODAY I AM GRATEFUL FOR...

PERSONAL HIGH FIVES (WINS)

HOW DID YOU EXPRESS GRATITUDE TODAY?

WHAT DID YOU GIVE TODAY THAT FILLED YOUR HEART?

TODAY I AM GRATEFUL FOR...

PERSONAL HIGH FIVES (WINS)

HOW DID YOU EXPRESS GRATITUDE TODAY?

WHAT HEALTH CARE PRODUCT ARE YOU MOST GRATEFUL FOR?

TODAY I AM GRATEFUL FOR...

PERSONAL HIGH FIVES (WINS)

HOW DID YOU EXPRESS GRATITUDE TODAY?

WHAT IS ONE THING THAT DIDN'T TURN OUT THE WAY YOU WANTED AND, IN HINDSIGHT, YOU ARE GRATEFUL?

TODAY I AM GRATEFUL FOR...

PERSONAL HIGH FIVES (WINS)

HOW DID YOU EXPRESS GRATITUDE TODAY?

WHAT BEVERAGE ARE YOU MOST GRATEFUL FOR TODAY?

"I take great joy and appreciation of the small things in life."

MARLA GENOVA

TODAY I AM GRATEFUL FOR...

PERSONAL HIGH FIVES (WINS)

HOW DID YOU EXPRESS GRATITUDE TODAY?

WHAT LEARNING OPPORTUNITY ARE YOU MOST GRATEFUL FOR TODAY?

TODAY I AM GRATEFUL FOR...

PERSONAL HIGH FIVES (WINS)

HOW DID YOU EXPRESS GRATITUDE TODAY?

WHAT ARE YOU GRATEFUL FOR THAT'S "OLD"?

TODAY I AM GRATEFUL FOR...

PERSONAL HIGH FIVES (WINS)

HOW DID YOU EXPRESS GRATITUDE TODAY?

WHAT IS SOMETHING INVISIBLE YOU ARE GRATEFUL FOR?

TODAY I AM GRATEFUL FOR...

PERSONAL HIGH FIVES (WINS)

HOW DID YOU EXPRESS GRATITUDE TODAY?

WHAT SOUND MADE YOU SMILE TODAY?

TODAY I AM GRATEFUL FOR...

PERSONAL HIGH FIVES (WINS)

HOW DID YOU EXPRESS GRATITUDE TODAY?

WHAT CHANGE ARE YOU MOST GRATEFUL FOR?

TODAY I AM GRATEFUL FOR...

PERSONAL HIGH FIVES (WINS)

HOW DID YOU EXPRESS GRATITUDE TODAY?

WHAT MAKES YOU FEEL RICH?

"Gratitude can be found in both small moments and grand gestures."

JULIE BLACKBURN

TODAY I AM GRATEFUL FOR...

PERSONAL HIGH FIVES (WINS)

HOW DID YOU EXPRESS GRATITUDE TODAY?

WHAT FLOWERS MAKE YOU FEEL JOYFUL?

TODAY I AM GRATEFUL FOR...

PERSONAL HIGH FIVES (WINS)

HOW DID YOU EXPRESS GRATITUDE TODAY?

WHAT NEW IDEA ARE YOU GRATEFUL FOR?

TODAY I AM GRATEFUL FOR...

PERSONAL HIGH FIVES (WINS)

HOW DID YOU EXPRESS GRATITUDE TODAY?

WHAT COMPROMISE ARE YOU GRATEFUL FOR TODAY?

TODAY I AM GRATEFUL FOR...

PERSONAL HIGH FIVES (WINS)

HOW DID YOU EXPRESS GRATITUDE TODAY?

WHO ARE YOU PROUD OF TODAY?

TODAY I AM GRATEFUL FOR...

PERSONAL HIGH FIVES (WINS)

HOW DID YOU EXPRESS GRATITUDE TODAY?

WHAT ARE YOU MOST GRATEFUL FOR ABOUT YOUR PHYSICAL SURROUNDINGS?

"I am being grateful when I engage my inner capacity for empathy and compassion."

MARCUS ALEXANDER

TODAY I AM GRATEFUL FOR...

PERSONAL HIGH FIVES (WINS)

HOW DID YOU EXPRESS GRATITUDE TODAY?

WHAT ACT OF LOVE ARE YOU MOST GRATEFUL FOR TODAY?

TODAY I AM GRATEFUL FOR...

PERSONAL HIGH FIVES (WINS)

HOW DID YOU EXPRESS GRATITUDE TODAY?

WHAT SEEMINGLY SILLY THING ARE YOU GRATEFUL FOR TODAY?

TODAY I AM GRATEFUL FOR...

PERSONAL HIGH FIVES (WINS)

HOW DID YOU EXPRESS GRATITUDE TODAY?

WHAT DID YOU READ TODAY THAT YOU ARE GRATEFUL FOR?

TODAY I AM GRATEFUL FOR...

PERSONAL HIGH FIVES (WINS)

HOW DID YOU EXPRESS GRATITUDE TODAY?

WHAT MISTAKE ARE YOU MOST GRATEFUL FOR?

TODAY I AM GRATEFUL FOR...

PERSONAL HIGH FIVES (WINS)

HOW DID YOU EXPRESS GRATITUDE TODAY?

WHAT SMELL MADE YOU HAPPY TODAY?

TODAY I AM GRATEFUL FOR…

PERSONAL HIGH FIVES (WINS)

HOW DID YOU EXPRESS GRATITUDE TODAY?

WHAT ANIMAL ARE YOU MOST GRATEFUL FOR TODAY?

"I often express gratitude for things that seem not to warrant it because they are the greatest opportunities for learning and growing."

DIANE MEYER LOWMAN

TODAY I AM GRATEFUL FOR...

PERSONAL HIGH FIVES (WINS)

HOW DID YOU EXPRESS GRATITUDE TODAY?

WHAT LESSON IN SCHOOL ARE YOU MOST GRATEFUL FOR?

TODAY I AM GRATEFUL FOR...

PERSONAL HIGH FIVES (WINS)

HOW DID YOU EXPRESS GRATITUDE TODAY?

WHAT CHILDHOOD FRIENDSHIP ARE YOU MOST GRATEFUL FOR?

TODAY I AM GRATEFUL FOR...

PERSONAL HIGH FIVES (WINS)

HOW DID YOU EXPRESS GRATITUDE TODAY?

HOW DID YOU CELEBRATE TODAY?

TODAY I AM GRATEFUL FOR...

PERSONAL HIGH FIVES (WINS)

HOW DID YOU EXPRESS GRATITUDE TODAY?

WHOSE SMILE MADE YOUR DAY?

TODAY I AM GRATEFUL FOR...

PERSONAL HIGH FIVES (WINS)

HOW DID YOU EXPRESS GRATITUDE TODAY?

WHAT MAKES YOU FEEL AT PEACE?

"Intentional, enduring awareness for all that is good has helped reframe life's everyday little miracles for what they are. Miracles!"

LESLIE FORDE

TODAY I AM GRATEFUL FOR...

PERSONAL HIGH FIVES (WINS)

HOW DID YOU EXPRESS GRATITUDE TODAY?

WHAT'S THE MOST BEAUTIFUL PLACE YOU'VE EVER VISITED?

TODAY I AM GRATEFUL FOR...

PERSONAL HIGH FIVES (WINS)

HOW DID YOU EXPRESS GRATITUDE TODAY?

WHAT COMPLIMENT DID YOU GIVE TODAY?

TODAY I AM GRATEFUL FOR...

PERSONAL HIGH FIVES (WINS)

HOW DID YOU EXPRESS GRATITUDE TODAY?

WHAT CHAOS ARE YOU GRATEFUL FOR TODAY?

TODAY I AM GRATEFUL FOR...

PERSONAL HIGH FIVES (WINS)

HOW DID YOU EXPRESS GRATITUDE TODAY?

WHAT MADE YOU TRULY FEEL GOOD TODAY?

TODAY I AM GRATEFUL FOR...

PERSONAL HIGH FIVES (WINS)

HOW DID YOU EXPRESS GRATITUDE TODAY?

WHAT BOOK ARE YOU MOST GRATEFUL FOR?

TODAY I AM GRATEFUL FOR...

PERSONAL HIGH FIVES (WINS)

HOW DID YOU EXPRESS GRATITUDE TODAY?

WHAT OUTDOOR ACTIVITY ARE YOU MOST GRATEFUL FOR?

"Gratitude has helped me lean into the parts of my life that I truly love and use them as a touchstone to remember how many things are worth connecting to."

LAKAY CORNELL

TODAY I AM GRATEFUL FOR...

PERSONAL HIGH FIVES (WINS)

HOW DID YOU EXPRESS GRATITUDE TODAY?

WHAT GIFT DO YOU HAVE TO GIVE THE WORLD?

TODAY I AM GRATEFUL FOR...

PERSONAL HIGH FIVES (WINS)

HOW DID YOU EXPRESS GRATITUDE TODAY?

WHAT IS THE BEST GIFT YOU'VE EVER RECEIVED?

TODAY I AM GRATEFUL FOR...

PERSONAL HIGH FIVES (WINS)

HOW DID YOU EXPRESS GRATITUDE TODAY?

WHAT DREAM KEEPS YOU GOING?

TODAY I AM GRATEFUL FOR...

PERSONAL HIGH FIVES (WINS)

HOW DID YOU EXPRESS GRATITUDE TODAY?

WHAT IS ONE LITTLE THING YOU ENJOYED THAT TURNED OUT TO BE A BIG THING?

TODAY I AM GRATEFUL FOR...

PERSONAL HIGH FIVES (WINS)

HOW DID YOU EXPRESS GRATITUDE TODAY?

WHAT DO YOU TAKE PLEASURE IN THAT MOST PEOPLE MIGHT NOT?

"When we feel genuine appreciation for every little and big thing in our lives, then the Universe responds with more to be grateful for."

NATALIE SAGER

TODAY I AM GRATEFUL FOR...

PERSONAL HIGH FIVES (WINS)

HOW DID YOU EXPRESS GRATITUDE TODAY?

HOW DID YOU ENJOY "WASTED" TIME TODAY?

TODAY I AM GRATEFUL FOR...

PERSONAL HIGH FIVES (WINS)

HOW DID YOU EXPRESS GRATITUDE TODAY?

WHAT CURRENT OR NEW FRIENDSHIP ARE YOU MOST GRATEFUL FOR?

TODAY I AM GRATEFUL FOR...

PERSONAL HIGH FIVES (WINS)

HOW DID YOU EXPRESS GRATITUDE TODAY?

WHAT CHARITABLE ORGANIZATION ARE YOU MOST GRATEFUL FOR TODAY?

TODAY I AM GRATEFUL FOR...

PERSONAL HIGH FIVES (WINS)

HOW DID YOU EXPRESS GRATITUDE TODAY?

WHAT TEACHER FROM YOUR PAST ARE YOU MOST GRATEFUL FOR TODAY?

TODAY I AM GRATEFUL FOR…

PERSONAL HIGH FIVES (WINS)

HOW DID YOU EXPRESS GRATITUDE TODAY?

HOW DID YOU EXPERIENCE JOY TODAY?

TODAY I AM GRATEFUL FOR...

PERSONAL HIGH FIVES (WINS)

HOW DID YOU EXPRESS GRATITUDE TODAY?

HOW DID YOUR FAMILY MAKE YOU HAPPY TODAY?

"In order to cultivate gratitude we must learn presence, acceptance, and trust."

KELSEY SPERL

TODAY I AM GRATEFUL FOR...

PERSONAL HIGH FIVES (WINS)

HOW DID YOU EXPRESS GRATITUDE TODAY?

WHAT SMALL COMFORT DID YOU EXPERIENCE TODAY?

TODAY I AM GRATEFUL FOR...

PERSONAL HIGH FIVES (WINS)

HOW DID YOU EXPRESS GRATITUDE TODAY?

WHAT DID YOU DO TODAY THAT FELT GREAT?

TODAY I AM GRATEFUL FOR...

PERSONAL HIGH FIVES (WINS)

HOW DID YOU EXPRESS GRATITUDE TODAY?

WHAT ARE YOU CURIOUS ABOUT TODAY?

TODAY I AM GRATEFUL FOR...

PERSONAL HIGH FIVES (WINS)

HOW DID YOU EXPRESS GRATITUDE TODAY?

WHAT LOCAL RESOURCES ARE YOU MOST GRATEFUL FOR?

TODAY I AM GRATEFUL FOR...

PERSONAL HIGH FIVES (WINS)

HOW DID YOU EXPRESS GRATITUDE TODAY?

WHAT DID YOU LEARN ABOUT YOURSELF TODAY?

"Gratitude is recognizing the ways in which you're blessed and carrying those blessings forward."

JOHN HOWARD

TODAY I AM GRATEFUL FOR...

PERSONAL HIGH FIVES (WINS)

HOW DID YOU EXPRESS GRATITUDE TODAY?

HOW WERE YOU COURAGEOUS TODAY?

TODAY I AM GRATEFUL FOR...

PERSONAL HIGH FIVES (WINS)

HOW DID YOU EXPRESS GRATITUDE TODAY?

USE ONE BEAUTIFUL WORD TO DESCRIBE YOURSELF.

TODAY I AM GRATEFUL FOR...

PERSONAL HIGH FIVES (WINS)

HOW DID YOU EXPRESS GRATITUDE TODAY?

WHAT DO YOU LOVE ABOUT YOURSELF?

TODAY I AM GRATEFUL FOR...

PERSONAL HIGH FIVES (WINS)

HOW DID YOU EXPRESS GRATITUDE TODAY?

WHAT WARMED YOUR HEART TODAY?

TODAY I AM GRATEFUL FOR...

PERSONAL HIGH FIVES (WINS)

HOW DID YOU EXPRESS GRATITUDE TODAY?

HOW DID YOU REWARD YOURSELF TODAY?

TODAY I AM GRATEFUL FOR...

PERSONAL HIGH FIVES (WINS)

HOW DID YOU EXPRESS GRATITUDE TODAY?

WHAT MADE YOU SMILE TODAY?

"In ordinary life, we hardly realize that we receive a great deal more than we give, and that it is only with gratitude that life becomes rich."

DIETRICH BONHOEFFER

TODAY I AM GRATEFUL FOR...

PERSONAL HIGH FIVES (WINS)

HOW DID YOU EXPRESS GRATITUDE TODAY?

WHAT DIFFICULTY HAVE YOU RECENTLY OVERCOME?

TODAY I AM GRATEFUL FOR...

PERSONAL HIGH FIVES (WINS)

HOW DID YOU EXPRESS GRATITUDE TODAY?

WHO DO YOU WANT TO CELEBRATE TODAY?

TODAY I AM GRATEFUL FOR...

PERSONAL HIGH FIVES (WINS)

HOW DID YOU EXPRESS GRATITUDE TODAY?

WHAT CHALLENGE ARE YOU MOST GRATEFUL FOR?

TODAY I AM GRATEFUL FOR...

PERSONAL HIGH FIVES (WINS)

HOW DID YOU EXPRESS GRATITUDE TODAY?

WHAT SOUND MOST COMFORTS YOU?

TODAY I AM GRATEFUL FOR...

PERSONAL HIGH FIVES (WINS)

HOW DID YOU EXPRESS GRATITUDE TODAY?

WHAT FREE THING ARE YOU MOST GRATEFUL FOR?

"Gratitude turns what we have into enough and more."

MELODY BEATTIE

TODAY I AM GRATEFUL FOR...

PERSONAL HIGH FIVES (WINS)

HOW DID YOU EXPRESS GRATITUDE TODAY?

HOW DID YOU INVEST IN YOURSELF TODAY?

TODAY I AM GRATEFUL FOR...

PERSONAL HIGH FIVES (WINS)

HOW DID YOU EXPRESS GRATITUDE TODAY?

WHAT NEW THING ARE YOU EXCITED TO TRY?

TODAY I AM GRATEFUL FOR...

PERSONAL HIGH FIVES (WINS)

HOW DID YOU EXPRESS GRATITUDE TODAY?

WHAT ELEMENT OF THE OUTSIDE ARE YOU MOST GRATEFUL FOR?

TODAY I AM GRATEFUL FOR...

PERSONAL HIGH FIVES (WINS)

HOW DID YOU EXPRESS GRATITUDE TODAY?

WHAT HAVE YOU ACHIEVED THAT YOU NEVER THOUGHT POSSIBLE?

TODAY I AM GRATEFUL FOR...

PERSONAL HIGH FIVES (WINS)

HOW DID YOU EXPRESS GRATITUDE TODAY?

WHAT DID YOU CELEBRATE TODAY?

TODAY I AM GRATEFUL FOR...

PERSONAL HIGH FIVES (WINS)

HOW DID YOU EXPRESS GRATITUDE TODAY?

WHAT COMPLIMENT DID YOU RECEIVE TODAY?

"I am grateful for what I am and have. My thanksgiving is perpetual."

HENRY DAVID THOREAU

TODAY I AM GRATEFUL FOR...

PERSONAL HIGH FIVES (WINS)

HOW DID YOU EXPRESS GRATITUDE TODAY?

WHO MADE A BIG DIFFERENCE IN YOUR LIFE TODAY?

TODAY I AM GRATEFUL FOR...

PERSONAL HIGH FIVES (WINS)

HOW DID YOU EXPRESS GRATITUDE TODAY?

WHOSE LIFE DID YOU MAKE A DIFFERENCE IN TODAY?

TODAY I AM GRATEFUL FOR...

PERSONAL HIGH FIVES (WINS)

HOW DID YOU EXPRESS GRATITUDE TODAY?

WHO WOULD YOU LIKE TO THANK TODAY?

TODAY I AM GRATEFUL FOR...

PERSONAL HIGH FIVES (WINS)

HOW DID YOU EXPRESS GRATITUDE TODAY?

WHAT MADE YOU FEEL ALIVE TODAY?

TODAY I AM GRATEFUL FOR...

PERSONAL HIGH FIVES (WINS)

HOW DID YOU EXPRESS GRATITUDE TODAY?

WHAT DID YOU HAPPILY SAY YES TO TODAY?

"Gratitude is the bridge between the positive things in our lives. Without that bridge, we can't move forward."

AKIRA AK

TODAY I AM GRATEFUL FOR...

PERSONAL HIGH FIVES (WINS)

HOW DID YOU EXPRESS GRATITUDE TODAY?

WHAT ARE YOU MOST GRATEFUL FOR IN THE FALL?

TODAY I AM GRATEFUL FOR...

PERSONAL HIGH FIVES (WINS)

HOW DID YOU EXPRESS GRATITUDE TODAY?

WHAT IS YOUR FAVORITE CHILDHOOD MEMORY?

TODAY I AM GRATEFUL FOR...

PERSONAL HIGH FIVES (WINS)

HOW DID YOU EXPRESS GRATITUDE TODAY?

WHAT MAKES YOU FEEL EMPOWERED?

TODAY I AM GRATEFUL FOR...

PERSONAL HIGH FIVES (WINS)

HOW DID YOU EXPRESS GRATITUDE TODAY?

WHAT GUILTY PLEASURE ARE YOU MOST GRATEFUL FOR?

TODAY I AM GRATEFUL FOR...

PERSONAL HIGH FIVES (WINS)

HOW DID YOU EXPRESS GRATITUDE TODAY?

HOW DID YOU CHANGE YOUR MIND TODAY?

TODAY I AM GRATEFUL FOR...

PERSONAL HIGH FIVES (WINS)

HOW DID YOU EXPRESS GRATITUDE TODAY?

WHAT DAILY RITUAL IS MOST POWERFUL FOR YOU?

"No one who achieves success does so without the help of others. The wise and confident acknowledge this help with gratitude."

ALFRED NORTH WHITEHEAD

TODAY I AM GRATEFUL FOR...

PERSONAL HIGH FIVES (WINS)

HOW DID YOU EXPRESS GRATITUDE TODAY?

WHAT'S YOUR FAVORITE WAY TO USE YOUR BODY?

TODAY I AM GRATEFUL FOR...

PERSONAL HIGH FIVES (WINS)

HOW DID YOU EXPRESS GRATITUDE TODAY?

WHAT'S THE BEST GIFT YOU'VE EVER GIVEN?

TODAY I AM GRATEFUL FOR...

PERSONAL HIGH FIVES (WINS)

HOW DID YOU EXPRESS GRATITUDE TODAY?

WHAT "THANK YOU" WAS THE MOST MEANINGFUL TO YOU?

TODAY I AM GRATEFUL FOR...

PERSONAL HIGH FIVES (WINS)

HOW DID YOU EXPRESS GRATITUDE TODAY?

WHAT DO YOU ENJOY MOST ABOUT GOING FOR A WALK?

TODAY I AM GRATEFUL FOR...

PERSONAL HIGH FIVES (WINS)

HOW DID YOU EXPRESS GRATITUDE TODAY?

WHAT IS YOUR FAVORITE WAY TO SPOIL YOURSELF?

"Bounty isn't just gathering more; it's appreciating what we have and knowing what we truly need."

LEIGH SCHWAB

TODAY I AM GRATEFUL FOR...

PERSONAL HIGH FIVES (WINS)

HOW DID YOU EXPRESS GRATITUDE TODAY?

WHAT SURPRISE ARE YOU GRATEFUL FOR?

TODAY I AM GRATEFUL FOR...

PERSONAL HIGH FIVES (WINS)

HOW DID YOU EXPRESS GRATITUDE TODAY?

WHAT NEW DOOR OPENED FOR YOU TODAY?

TODAY I AM GRATEFUL FOR...

PERSONAL HIGH FIVES (WINS)

HOW DID YOU EXPRESS GRATITUDE TODAY?

WHAT MADE YOU FEEL CONNECTED TODAY?

TODAY I AM GRATEFUL FOR...

PERSONAL HIGH FIVES (WINS)

HOW DID YOU EXPRESS GRATITUDE TODAY?

WHAT DELIGHTED YOU TODAY?

TODAY I AM GRATEFUL FOR…

PERSONAL HIGH FIVES (WINS)

HOW DID YOU EXPRESS GRATITUDE TODAY?

HOW DID YOU COME THROUGH FOR SOMEONE ELSE TODAY?

TODAY I AM GRATEFUL FOR...

PERSONAL HIGH FIVES (WINS)

HOW DID YOU EXPRESS GRATITUDE TODAY?

WHAT NEW EXPERIENCE ARE YOU GRATEFUL FOR TODAY?

"Enjoy every moment of the journey, and appreciate where you are at this moment instead of always focusing on how far you have to go."

MANDY HALE

TODAY'S DATE _____ / _____ / _____

TODAY I AM GRATEFUL FOR...

PERSONAL HIGH FIVES (WINS)

HOW DID YOU EXPRESS GRATITUDE TODAY?

WHO DID YOU FORGIVE TODAY?

TODAY I AM GRATEFUL FOR...

PERSONAL HIGH FIVES (WINS)

HOW DID YOU EXPRESS GRATITUDE TODAY?

WHAT DID YOU LET GO OF TODAY?

TODAY I AM GRATEFUL FOR...

PERSONAL HIGH FIVES (WINS)

HOW DID YOU EXPRESS GRATITUDE TODAY?

WHAT RANDOM ACT OF KINDNESS DID YOU EXPERIENCE TODAY?

TODAY I AM GRATEFUL FOR...

PERSONAL HIGH FIVES (WINS)

HOW DID YOU EXPRESS GRATITUDE TODAY?

WHAT ARE YOU MOST GRATEFUL FOR IN THE WINTER?

TODAY I AM GRATEFUL FOR...

PERSONAL HIGH FIVES (WINS)

HOW DID YOU EXPRESS GRATITUDE TODAY?

WHAT ARE YOU PASSIONATE ABOUT TODAY?

"I express gratitude to myself by staying aligned in my emotional, physical, mental, and spiritual center, and making myself a priority so that I can continue on my path and purpose."

SUPNA SHAH

TODAY I AM GRATEFUL FOR...

PERSONAL HIGH FIVES (WINS)

HOW DID YOU EXPRESS GRATITUDE TODAY?

HOW DID WORK BECOME PLAY TODAY?

TODAY I AM GRATEFUL FOR...

PERSONAL HIGH FIVES (WINS)

HOW DID YOU EXPRESS GRATITUDE TODAY?

WHAT SOOTHED YOU TODAY?

TODAY I AM GRATEFUL FOR...

PERSONAL HIGH FIVES (WINS)

HOW DID YOU EXPRESS GRATITUDE TODAY?

WHAT PLEASURE DID YOU GIVE TODAY?

TODAY I AM GRATEFUL FOR...

PERSONAL HIGH FIVES (WINS)

HOW DID YOU EXPRESS GRATITUDE TODAY?

HOW DID YOU PLAY TODAY?

TODAY I AM GRATEFUL FOR...

PERSONAL HIGH FIVES (WINS)

HOW DID YOU EXPRESS GRATITUDE TODAY?

HOW DID YOU SERVE OTHERS TODAY?

TODAY I AM GRATEFUL FOR...

PERSONAL HIGH FIVES (WINS)

HOW DID YOU EXPRESS GRATITUDE TODAY?

WHAT "UNIMPORTANT" THING ARE YOU MOST GRATEFUL FOR TODAY?

"When I approach my day full of gratitude, I come into it focused on what's working and I expect more good things to come. Practicing gratitude is one of the closest things to a 'happy pill' I've ever found."

CHRISTINE MCALISTER

TODAY I AM GRATEFUL FOR...

PERSONAL HIGH FIVES (WINS)

HOW DID YOU EXPRESS GRATITUDE TODAY?

WHAT MADE YOU CHEERFUL TODAY?

TODAY I AM GRATEFUL FOR...

PERSONAL HIGH FIVES (WINS)

HOW DID YOU EXPRESS GRATITUDE TODAY?

WHAT ARE YOU MOST GRATEFUL FOR IN THE SUMMER?

TODAY I AM GRATEFUL FOR...

PERSONAL HIGH FIVES (WINS)

HOW DID YOU EXPRESS GRATITUDE TODAY?

WHAT ARE YOU MOST GRATEFUL FOR GIVING TODAY?

TODAY I AM GRATEFUL FOR...

PERSONAL HIGH FIVES (WINS)

HOW DID YOU EXPRESS GRATITUDE TODAY?

WHAT NON-TANGIBLE THING ARE YOU MOST GRATEFUL FOR TODAY?

"Never let the things you want make you forget the things you have."

SANCHITA PANDEY

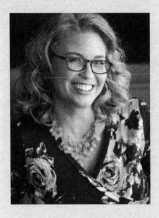

About the Author

Heather Vickery is an award-winning business owner and Success Coach, with over 20 years of experience and Positive Psychology certification from the University of Pennsylvania. She leverages her entrepreneurial skills and expertise to coach individuals towards greater personal and professional fulfillment. A celebrated public speaker, Heather inspires audiences and empowers attendees with the tools they need to live bold and successful lives through creating balance with time management, as well as countless systems, strategies, and boundaries. Heather is a mom of four, dedicated community member, and a fierce advocate for social justice. She's also the executive producer and host of the Brave Files podcast.

    @vickeryandco

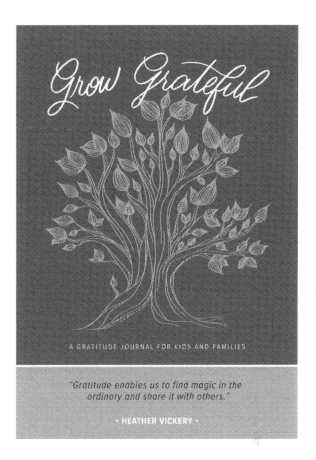

Give your kids the gift of gratitude and help them develop skills for happiness and wellbeing.

"The energy of gratitude is a powerful, life-changing practice you must master when you're hoping to live a more amazing, joyful, abundant life. This book is not only written with that energy, it teaches this magical practice to you and your kids, in a simple, beautiful way. Growing Grateful is a gift you'll always feel incredible about giving."

- **Laura Di Franco, MPT**, *Owner of Brave Healer Productions*

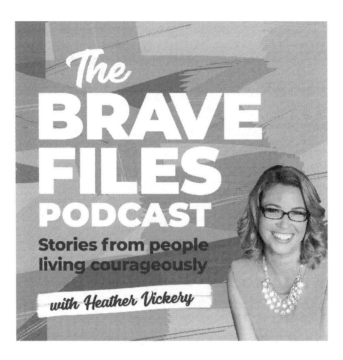

When we choose bravely, in every possible way, our lives are infinitely better.

Tune in each week for a dose of inspiration from a guest who's living courageously.

Inspiration. Motivation. Human Connection.

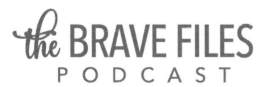

Find us on Apple Podcast, Spotify, Stitcher, Google and anywhere you enjoy podcasts.

Made in the USA
Monee, IL
12 October 2020